The CURSE

"BREAKING GENERATIONAL CURSE"

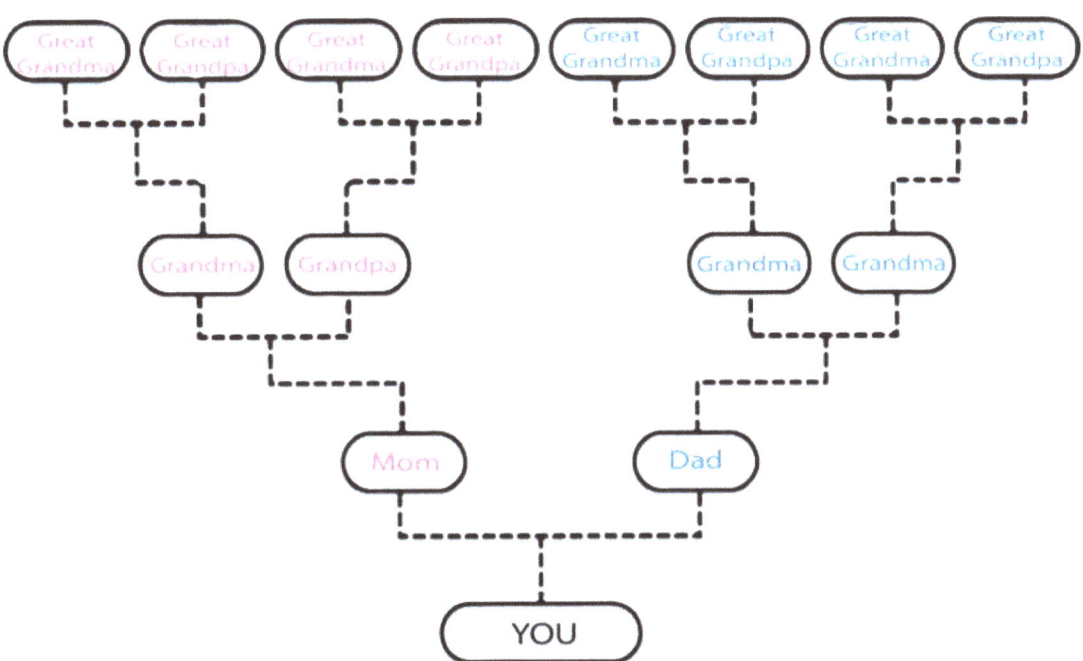

BY

TIMOTHY MITCHELL

Introduction

Do you suffer from the same physical illnesses as your family members? Are your behaviors destructive and appear impossible to correct or extinguish? Do you notice the same destructive behavioral patterns in your family members from one generation to the next? If you answered yes to any of these questions, you might be experiencing a generational curse. A generational curse is simply any ailment of the mind, body, and spirit resulting from negative behavioral patterns passed down throughout several generations. Some examples of generational curses are addictions (i.e., drug/alcohol, sex), mental illnesses (depression, schizophrenia, bipolar depression), physical illnesses (hypertension, heart disease, cancer), and even poverty, to name a few. To deal with a generational curse and eradicate it, one must understand the origin and the dimensions of a generational curse.

Generational curses are applied and maintained on three levels. They are the genetic, environmental, and supernatural levels. Because these strongholds are three-dimensional, it may be challenging to overcome them. The first is the genetic or biological level. It is essential to understand that generational curses began with the fall of man in the Garden of Eden, and because of that, "we were born into sin and shaped in iniquity." Although we are made in the image of God and are genetically predisposed to behave as He would, we adapted a sinful nature because of the sin of Adam and Eve.

An example of a generational curse on the genetic level is a physical illness or disease that plagues families for generations. Medical studies indicate a genetic component for many diseases such as diabetes, heart disease, and certain cancers. That is the very reason medical professionals request information about one's family history and lifestyle when seeking treatment. Medical professionals understand that lifestyles or behaviors that result in illnesses will be passed down throughout several generations.

The second level on which a generational curse is maintained is through our environment. It must be understood that we acquire many of our behaviors, good and bad, from our families of origin. Remember, most destructive habits or lifestyles result from learned behavioral patterns passed down from one generation to the next. We absorb a lot of information about our world from our families of origin, and we relate to others in our world based on that information. Examples of generational curses on the environmental level are poverty, broken relationships, and divorces. Sociological studies have repeatedly proven that families of low socioeconomic classes have tendencies to remain in poverty for several generations. This is because of a consistent lack of exposure to environments that foster educational and financial advancement. Research on marriage and family suggests that destructive behaviors taught within each spouse's family of origin contribute to the dissolution of marriages.

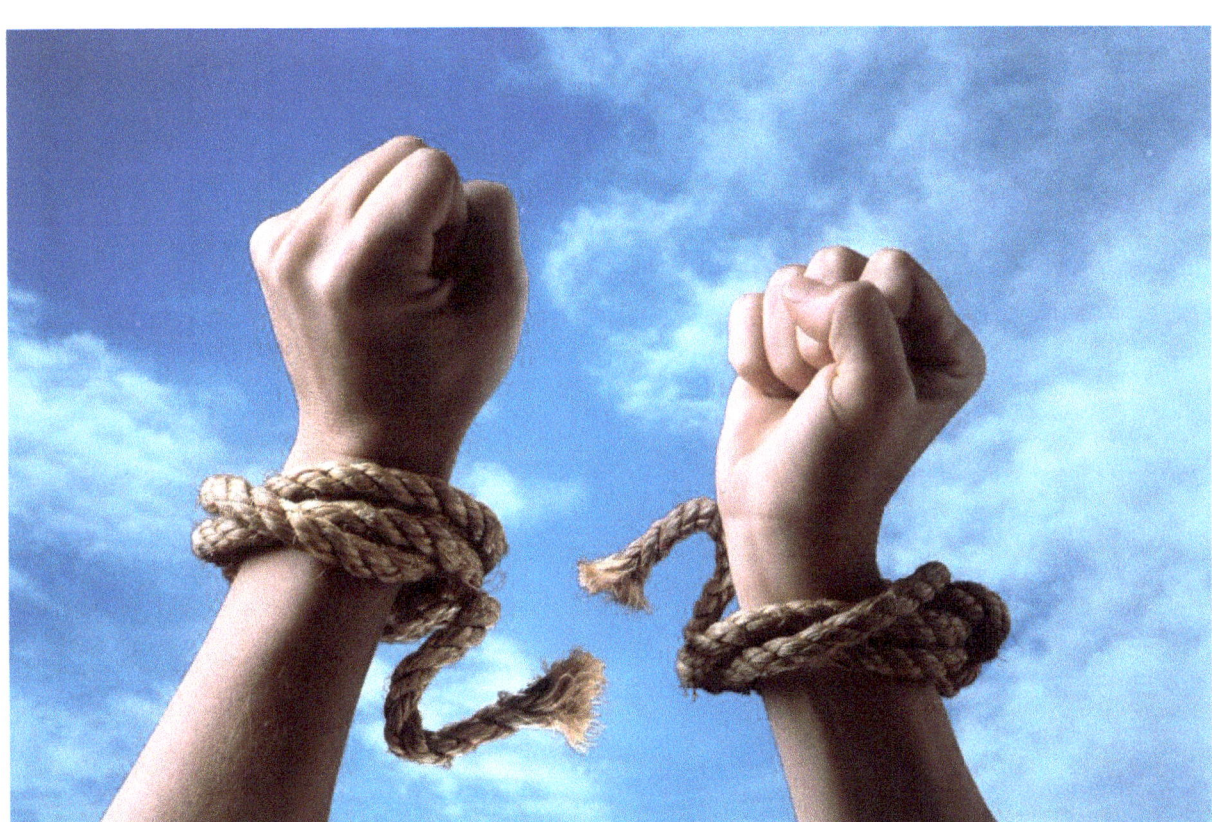

What Is Generational Curse?

These are recurring issues that the enemy uses to steal, kill, and destroy. They are passed down from one generation to another. The Bible says God punishes the children for their parents' sins to the third and fourth generations. (Exodus 20:5)

Examples of generational curses include divorce, hereditary sickness, sexual immorality, poverty, depression, child abuse, and perversion. Understand that we don't struggle with curses when there is no cause (Proverbs 26:4). When family members sin, they give access to evil spirits who wreak havoc in our lives through generational curses.

But how can a person identify generational curses?

Signs Of Generational Curses

We need to know the signs of generational curses. That way, we can identify the types of courses that they may be running in our family: However, we should not be quick to point out some things as generational curses. We should ask God to show us which curses are in our family lines during our prayer time.

Below are some of the most common signs of generational curses. As you go through this list, ask the Holy Spirit to give you revelation. The Spirit of the Lord is the only one who knows deep spiritual matters.

- ❖ **Fear/Emotional instability**

In Deuteronomy 28:28, God says that he will strike those who disobey him with madness, blindness, and confusion. Meaning that insanity, irrational behavior, foolishness, confusion, and indecision may be generational curses.

When people with this generational curse are overcome by fear or emotions they:

- Make foolish decisions and do crazy, self-destructive things.
- Have a continual struggle, frustration, and internal warfare.

Another thing to note about this generational curse is people who have it struggle with double-mindedness. They struggle to align their lives with the word of God. When they try to renew their minds, they experience a lot of warfare. And this discourages them from abiding in the word of God.

Those with this generational curse should know that they're children of God saved by grace. Remember that your heavenly Father is not the author of confusion. So all these things are not your portion.

❖ **Hereditary illnesses**

It almost sounds normal for family members to have the same disease in this current world. Evil seems familiar to us that we may fail to see some things as generational curses. Sickness is one of those things that we can easily overlook. The generational curse of hereditary illness releases sickness of all kinds.

You may find that people struggle or die from one particular disease in a family. Do not look at it lightly or from a scientific point of view alone. Maybe someone in your family line opened up doors for the spirit behind hereditary sickness.

❖ **Chronic wounds**

Deuteronomy 28:27, God told the Israelites that he would attack them with botches of Egypt. That is, if they disobeyed him. But what are botches, you may ask? These are boils or open sores. People with chronic wounds, that is, wounds that cannot heal, experience these. This curse attacks the top of a person's head, the feet' soles, and the legs.

❖ Barrenness and fertility problems

Ever heard someone call menstrual problems 'the curse'? Well, some of the folklore we know has its roots in biblical tradition. So some menstrual problems may be a result of curses.

The word says that cursed shall be the fruit of thy body (Deuteronomy 28:18). The word body in this text is the same as the Hebrew word 'been,' which means womb, abdomen, or belly.

Now we all know that the womb is a reproductive organ. So barrenness and fertility problems can be a curse. The following are signs of this curse: hormonal problems, fibroids. Others include miscarriages, tumors, cysts, painful sex, PMS, cramps, and kidney stones.

These signs plague millions of women. This doesn't mean that all of them are under a curse. But some of them struggle with these signs because of curses. Men who manifest this curse struggle with impotence and erectile dysfunction.

❖ Family Struggles and Divorce

Do you know that America's divorce rate for first marriages is 50%, 67% for second marriages? And 74% for those that are in their third marriages? Sad, right? In Japan, the divorce rate is 27%, 10% in Singapore, and 1% in India.

Families with these curses struggle with family divides and battles, jailed children, divorce, and estranged relationships. Marital problems do not just affect parents; they also affect children.

Why? The sins of fathers are visited on their children (Deuteronomy 28: 32). Here are statistics of family problems to help us see how true and serious this is:

- Children from fatherless homes are estimated to be 1.2 million
- Those who are at home without parents supervision, that is, latchkey kids, are 1.8 million
- 36% of children grow up without their fathers.
- 75% of children in juvenile come from single-parent homes
- 63% of youths who commit suicide come from single-parent homes
- 70% of teenage pregnancies are from single-parent homes
- 75% of children doing drugs come from single-parent homes

❖ **Poverty**

Some families live in abject poverty. Whatever project they try always fails, and they always have financial struggles. It could be that their parents and great-grandparents also went through financial struggles, luck, and inability to produce. It is not that these people are lazy; it's just that whatever they try does not succeed.

Deuteronomy 28:17 says that cursed will be the kneading basket and stores of those who disobey God. The enemy usually stops the ability to produce wealth for people who struggle with this generational curse. Such people never have anything saved. Bill collectors always oppress them, and whatever little they produce is stolen by spoilers.

❖ **Debtors**

Families with this generational curse are always slaves to creditors because they're ever in debt (Deuteronomy 28:47-48). There are teachings out there that say not having is a blessing. But those teachings are wrong and misleading because God wants you to enjoy the fruits of your labor.

God wants us to have all that we need and plenty of left-over so that we can share with others (2 Corinthians 9:8). A person with this curse squanders and wastes their money, causing them to get further in debt and bondage. Get-rich schemes of all kinds easily influence them.

Generational Curse Of No Ambition Vision Or Direction

Do you know someone who has no intention or vision for their life? They have no set goals and are always going to and fro in life. These people always let the issues of life determine how they live. They go aimlessly through life and care less about tomorrow.

We need to have ambitions in life because we are God's stewards. None of us are here by accident. There are things God wants us to accomplish in this life. Having a vision, setting goals, and following God's direction will help you fulfill your purpose.

People with ambition have a strong desire to make a difference in life. They have dreams or aspirations to succeed. But people with the generational curse of lack of purpose are always negative in life. They are always full of lukewarmness, uncertainty, and apathy.

- ❖ **Bondage and slavery**

Individuals under the curse of bondage and slavery are easily manipulated and controlled. Some of them are controlled to the point of losing their identity. People under bondage cannot make decisions on their own. They have to get permission from their masters. In some cases, their masters may be controlling parents, husbands, lovers, cult leaders, and even pastors.

These people will look to other gods for protection and provision, not the Lord. They are full of idolatry, sensuality and are addicted to different forms of entertainment. They are bound to anything that separates them from the lordship of Jesus Christ.

Types Of Generational Curses

One of the dynamics that we need to be aware of in the deliverance ministry is generational curses. There is no one formula for these. But breakthroughs, deliverance, and healing happen in most people's lives when they are set free from strongholds and generational curses.

If a tree produces rotten fruits, chances are the roots are rotten. Generational curses are like bad roots beneath that produce rotten fruits in our lives. They need to be uprooted. We receive an inheritance from our parents by receiving a spiritual heritage from our family line.

Physical inheritance comes in traits and looks. At the same time, the spiritual inheritance comes in blessings and curses (Exodus 20:4-6).

Just so we're apparent generational curses do not mean that God charges children for the sins of their parents (Ezekiel 18:19-20). But the sins of our parents harm us as children. And they open doors for similar patterns of sin in our lives.

Parents are supposed to provide spiritual protection to their children. But when they walk in iniquity, sin, and idolatry, their children are left vulnerable to the enemy's attack.

Adam and Eve passed their sinful nature to their offspring. Similarly, our evil tendencies also pass on to our offspring if we do not repent.

Here are four types of curses that parents pass on to their children:

❖ Idolatry or Occult

When we worship any another thing except the one true living God, we practice idolatry. Idol worship is done in so many different ways. Some people worship physical idols like graven images and money. But there are also nonphysical things that people worship, like pride.

The Bible equates covetousness to idolatry (Ezekiel 14:3). Good things like your job, business, family, and entertainment can also become Idols in our hearts. We should always ascribe to God and worship him alone.

Occultism is another form of idolatry. People who engage in this activity seeks to gain things from evil spirits instead of God. There are so many different ways people practice occultism. But one common thing that people who practice occultism do is take oaths and curses. In some cases, they have to commit their children to the curses.

The iniquities of people who practice idolatry and occultism pass from one generation to another. Families with this generational curse experience overshadowing darkness over their lives, pain, destructive patterns. They struggle with unexplainable sickness and are always drawing themselves to spiritual darkness.

❖ Sinful patterns

Ever wondered why some families are prone to certain sins? For example, you may find families whose members are thieves or drug traffickers. It is easy to hear people calling such families cursed, and at times they are right. Various factors influence such families, and one of them is generational curses.

When sinful strongholds are not broken, they end up being passed down from one generation to another. For example, if there's a sexual sin pattern in the family, family members may struggle with sexual sin.

It could be that your parents always struggled with anger. And you're also struggling with uncontrollable anger. That could be a sign that it is a generational curse in your family.

Abraham lied to Pharaoh and Abimelech that Sarah was not his wife. Isaac did the same (Genesis 26:8-10). Jacob, Abraham's grandson, also used deception to get blessings from his Father, Isaac. We see a pattern of sin that was passed from one generation to another in this family.

So we are clear you should not blame your parents or previous generations for your own sinful choices. You need to take responsibility for your actions and repent when you sin. But it is still essential to find out generational curses in your family line.

When you've identified that something runs within the family line, and it's a generational curse, it'll be easy for you to understand why you keep doing certain things.

It'll also help you receive deliverance from sinful strongholds and any form of evil spirits that attach themselves to the stronghold. As such, we can begin to walk in the blessings of God. And when we conquer these sinful patterns, our children inherit our blessings.

❖ Faulty Mindsets and Destructive Behaviors

Just like sinful patterns, faulty mindsets and destructive behaviors can also be passed through generations. It could be that you've noticed cycles of harmful tendencies in your family line.

Maybe people in your family have been committing suicide or harming themselves. Or perhaps you come from a family of alcoholics and drug addicts. The enemy not only comes to steal, kill, and destroy, but he also wants to lay hold of individuals. And to establish strongholds in their family lines.

Destructive behaviors that are generational can be identified easily. But when it comes to faulty mindsets, it can be difficult to notice them. For example, a family can be struggling with the stronghold of legalism and traditionalism.

Since traditions may seem ordinary, it may be difficult for you to identify them as generational curses. But with the help of the Holy Spirit, you can identify this destructive behavior and be able to break it.

Other examples of faulty mindsets include skepticism, perfectionism, judgmental attitudes, and condemnation.

❖ Physical/ Mental Sickness

One of the things that doctors ask for before they perform specific procedures is your family's medical history. It's easy to assume that sickness results from our genes when the root cause is spiritual.

Yes, not every sickness is a result of a curse. But when you look at Deuteronomy 28, certain diseases and mental disorders are included in the curses list.

Examples of diseases that can pass through bloodlines are depression, anxiety, bipolar, miscarriages, cancer, and heart disease. It is not in God's plan for his children to be sick or struggle with a mental torment.

God wants to bless and heal us. That is why he gave up his only Son to die on the cross for us. If there is a disease in your family and a generational curse, do not get scared.

Instead, the knowledge of its existence should equip you. It becomes easy for us to receive healing and walk in divine health when we are fully equipped.

Why Are Generational Curses So Hard To Break?

Some people wonder why it is hard to break generational curses. Well, the truth is they are not exactly hard to break. Jesus has already won the battle at the cross. But most of us struggle to break them because of:

- ❖ **Wrong Teachings**

We need to be careful about what we see and hear. The word of God tells us to guard our hearts, and how do we do that? By guarding our eye and ear gates. When you feed on wrong teachings about breaking generational cycles, curses become hard to break.

Some people have been lied to that they need to do certain rituals to break curses. Others have been told they don't have to do anything. So they are torn between breaking these curses or doing nothing.

Yes, Jesus has won the battle, but that doesn't mean that we should not repent. Please only follow Bible-based teachings. Avoid anything that does not align with the word of God.

- **Ignorance**

Many of us struggle because we deal with issues of generational curses half haphazardly. We do not take time to find out what the Bible says about generational curses. We break them without taking the time to research our bloodlines. And hence end up praying amiss when breaking curses.

- **Fear**

A lot of information about spiritual warfare is flawed. The enemy is magnified, and God is presented as an angry God ready to punish his children. Yes, we have to take responsibility for our Christian walk. But we should never forget that we serve a merciful God. He leaves the ninety-nine to look for the one lost sheep.

Again it is not hard to break generational curses because Jesus took every curse on his body. We need to know that it takes time for many people to break generational curses. Here is why:

- **Generational curses are deep-rooted.**

Unlike other personal sins, generational curses are deep-rooted because they have been there from one generation to another. We must understand our family history and know our bloodlines to pray effectively. Finding all that information may take longer, primarily if we do not rely on the Holy Spirit.

How Do We Break Generational Curses?

Breaking Generational Curses

As we have already said, for someone to destroy these curses effectively, they need to know what kind of curses are in the family line. You cannot break generational curses in your strength. It would be best if you had the wisdom of the Holy Spirit. So ask God for wisdom and then follow these five steps when breaking generational cycles.

- ❖ **Surrender to God Wholeheartedly**

We are told in the word to submit to God, resist the devil, and he will flee (James 4:7). This means that it is by submitting to God that we can resist the enemy. And this, in turn, causes him to flee from us. But what does submission mean?

It means to submit your spirit, soul, and body to God and allow him to take over and reside in you. Submitting to God also means standing firm on his word.

And believing that he is faithful and more than able to defeat the enemy. Believe that Jesus has already defeated the enemy at the cross. So Satan has no power over you and the generations to come.

- ❖ **Confess the Iniquities of your Family and your Own**

You need to confess any known sin in your life. If there is some unknown sin in your life, God will reveal it to you so that you can repent and start living in his ways. Confess wholeheartedly the sins of your family, particularly the sins of your grandparents and parents.

The Bible tells us that if we confess our sins or the sins of our ancestors, God will forgive us. (Leviticus 26:40-42). By acknowledging our parents' and grandparents' sins, we know why the devil is attacking us.

It also makes you understand the adverse effects of sin. Hence, making it easy for you to understand the damaging effects of generational curses and live in the purposes of God.

With the Holy Spirit's help, we should list all known and unknown sins in our families. In your prayer time, declare every sin that your parents and grandparents have committed against God out loud. Then ask God to forgive your family and purify future generations.

❖ Forgive your Family Members

Many children from families who struggle with generational curses end up physically, mentally, and emotionally abused. And because of what they go through, they end up harboring hatred, anger, and guilt in their hearts.

To shut the doors of the enemy in your life, you need to forgive your parents and grandparents. Refusing to forgive will cause you to have an intense feeling of guilt, rage, and anger.

If these feelings are not dealt with early, they remain in the child's emotional setup and form mental strongholds. Strongholds give the devil access to torment and attack people.

❖ Separate yourself from Evil Soul Ties

Spiritual connections that take place between two people are what we call soul ties. Soul ties can be between parents and children, siblings, friends, and spouses. A soul tie can be healthy or unhealthy.

Unhealthy soul ties open up doors for generational curses so that one person becomes dominant. And that is usually the abusive person, while the other person becomes submissive.

The submissive person is usually hurt and abused. It's essential to break the evil soul tie between you and a dominant person in your life. Doing that enables you to break free from demonic attacks.

Note that demons get in the life of a person and feed on an unhealthy soul tie. It would help if you disconnected yourself from all kinds of disparaging soul ties before you start breaking any generational curse in your family life.

- **Break the generational Curse line**

When you complete the above step, and you'll be ready to break the curse line. Through curse lines, the devil and his demons gain access, function, and feed on. Now, you need to be saved first before going through these steps. The blood of Jesus Christ cleanses us from all sins, and through it, we trample over the enemy.

When breaking generational cycles, you need to use the weapons of warfare found in Ephesians 6:11-18.

Every believer has the spiritual authority to fight against the enemy and to trade on his powers. When breaking generational curses, you should stand firm in authority. And command every part of the curse in your family to be severed, removed, and broken in Jesus' name.

Now you may be wondering: what verses can I stand on? Which prayers can I pray to break these curses?

Scriptures About Breaking Generational Curse

Here are three scriptures that you can begin with:

- Christ redeemed us from the curse of the law by becoming a curse for us, for it is written: "Cursed is everyone who is hung on a pole." (Galatians 3:13)

- Yet you ask, 'Why does the son not share the guilt of his father?' Since the Son has done just and right and has been careful to keep all my decrees, he will surely live. (Ezekiel 18:19)

- Therefore, if anyone is in Christ, the new creation has come: The old has gone, the new is here! (2 Corinthians 5:17)

Prayer Points To Break Generational Curses

Here are five prayer points to start with if you don't know what prayers to pray against generational curses:

- Father God, reveal every generational curse in my bloodline from both sides of my family through your spirit in Jesus' name.

- Christ has redeemed me from the curse of the law by becoming a curse for me. Every demonic force reinforces generational curses in my life, leave my life alone, and go back to hell where you belong in Jesus' name.

- It is written the curse causeless shall not come (Proverbs 26:2), and it is also written whom the Son has set free is free indeed. Generational curse of sickness, I command you to leave my life right now and go back to hell where you belong. Jesus has set me free, so you have no cause in my life.

- It is written in 2 Corinthians 8:9 Jesus became poor so that I might become rich by his poverty. You curse poverty from both sides of my family; I declare that you are canceled from my life and future generations in Jesus' name.

- I cancel and nullify family curses that have been causing my life since childhood in Jesus' name. I purify my body and life with the blood of Jesus, the blood that speaks better things than the blood of Abel in Jesus' name.

Conclusion

Breaking generational curses is easy once you know the curses in your bloodline and how to break them. Some people, mostly some family members, will disagree with you about generational curses. And you are setting foundations for new changes in your life.

Make these people understand why you must break generational curses. Remember, God has not given us the spirit of fear, so deal with the curses in your bloodline without fear.

The devil may retaliate by attacking you differently, but stand firm in the word because whom the Son has set free is free indeed. Reject anything that conflicts with your identity in Christ.

Claim victory over yourself, your family, and generations to come. Remember, Jesus redeemed us from the curse of the law by becoming a curse himself. So freedom is your portion; you need to claim it now.

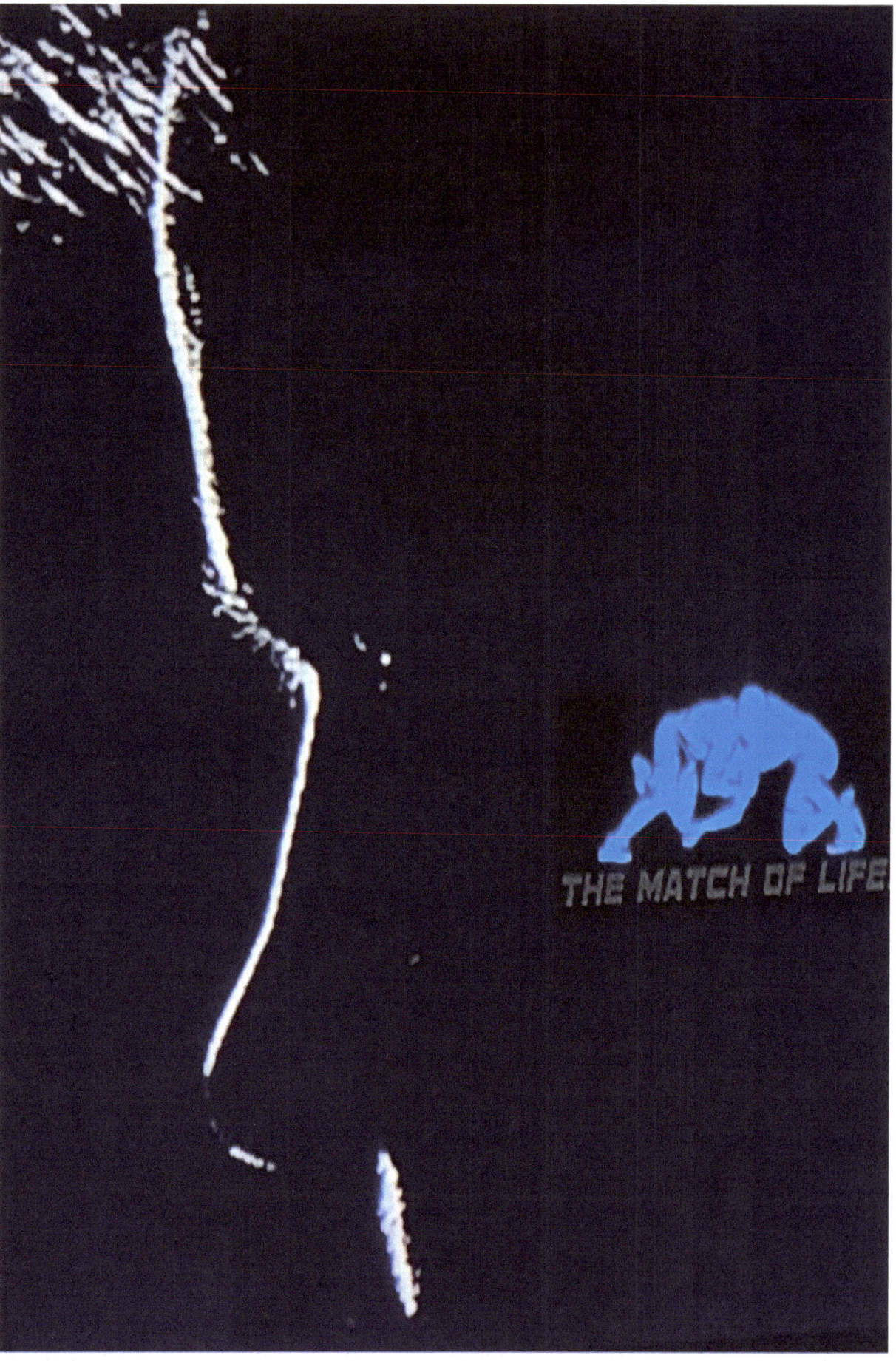

www.ingramcontent.com/pod-product-compliance
Lightning Source LLC
Chambersburg PA
CBHW061150010526
44118CB00026B/2935